What Does the Bible Say About Jesus?

What Does the Bible Say,
and Why Should I Care?

What's in the Bible About Jesus?

Paul E. Stroble

ABINGDON PRESS
NASHVILLE

WHAT'S IN THE BIBLE ABOUT JESUS?
by Paul Stroble

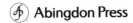 Abingdon Press

ISBN-13: 978-0-687-653836

Manufactured in the United States of America

08 09 10 11 12 13 14 15 16 17—10 9 8 7 6 5 4 3 2 1

CONTENTS

About the Writer vi

A Word From the Editor vii

A Word From the Writer ix

1. Who Is Jesus? 1

2. What Did Jesus Say? 21

3. What Did Jesus Do? 41

4. How Can We Respond

   to Jesus? 61

Appendix: Praying the Bible 83

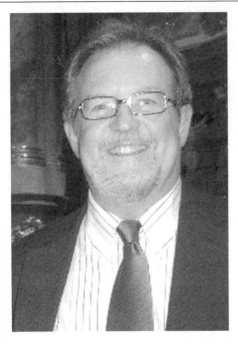

Paul Stroble is an elder of the Illinois Great Rivers Conference of The United Methodist Church. He studied at Greenville College, Yale Divinity School, and the University of Virginia. He has served as a parish pastor and volunteer leader at several churches and as a college teacher and seminary instructor. He currently teaches in the history department and Honors College at the University of Akron, where he earned an Excellence in Teaching Award. Paul is a writer-researcher for the United Methodist curriculum *FaithLink* and has written numerous articles, essays, poems, and curricular materials. Among his several books are *Paul and the Galatians, What Do Other Faiths Believe?* and *What About Religion and Science? A Study of Reason and Faith,* all for Abingdon Press, and *You Gave Me a Wide Place: Holy Places of Our Lives*, published by Upper Room Books. Paul has also written two books about his hometown, Vandalia, Illinois, and contributes to local historical efforts. Paul enjoys drawing, shopping in antique stores, and spending time with his wife, Dr. Beth Stroble, and their daughter, Emily.

About This Bible Study Series

Have you ever wondered what the Bible is all about? What's in it? Why is it so important for Christians? Is it relevant for people in the 21st century? Should I care about what's in the Bible? Why? What difference will it make in my life? The study series *What's in the Bible, and Why Should I Care?* offers opportunities for you to explore these questions and others by opening the Bible, reading it, prayerfully reflecting on what the Bible readings say, and making connections between the readings and your daily life. The series title points to the two essential features of meaningful Bible study: reading the Bible and applying it to your life. This unique and exciting Bible study series is designed to help you accomplish this two-fold purpose.

The books in *What's in the Bible, and Why Should I Care?* are designed to help you find relevance, hope, and meaning for your life even if you have little or no experience with the Bible. You will discover ways the Bible can help you with major questions you may have about the nature of God, how God relates to us, and how we can relate to God. Such questions continue to be relevant whether you are new to church life, a long-time member of church, or a seeker who is curious and wants to know more.

Whether you read a study book from this series on your own or with others in a Bible study group, you will experience benefits. You will gain confidence in reading the Bible as you learn how to use and study it. You will find meaning and hope in the people and teachings of the Bible. Most important, you will discover more about who God is and how God relates to you personally through the Bible.

What's in the Bible?

Obviously, we answer the question "What's in the Bible?" by reading it. As Christians, we understand that the stories of our faith come to us through this holy book. We view the Bible as the central document for all we believe and profess about God. It contains stories about those who came before us in the Christian faith, but it is more than a book of stories about them. The Bible tells us about God. It tells how a particular group of people in a particular part of the world over an extended period of time, inspired by God, understood and wrote about who God is and how God acted among them. It also tells what God expected from them. Its value and meaning reach to all people across all time—past, present, and future.

Why Should I Care?

Meaningful Bible study inspires people to live their lives according to God's will and way. As you read through the stories collected in the Bible, you will see again and again a just and merciful God who creates, loves, saves, and heals. You will see that God expects people, who are created in the image of God (Genesis 1), to live their lives as just and merciful people of God. You will discover that God empowers people to live according to God's way. You will learn that in spite of our sin, of our tendency to turn away from God and God's ways, God continues to love and save us. This theme emerges from and unifies all the books that have been brought together in the Holy Bible.

Christians believe that God's work of love and salvation finds confirmation and completion through the life, ministry, death, and resurrection of Jesus Christ. We accept God's free gift of love and salvation through Jesus Christ; and out of gratitude, we commit our lives to following him and living as he taught us to live. Empowered by God's Holy Spirit, we grow in faith, service, and love toward God and neighbor. I pray that this Bible study series will help you experience God's love and power in your daily life. I pray that it will help you grow in your faith and commitment to Jesus Christ.

Pamela Dilmore

How is your spiritual life right now? Do you feel close to God or far from God?

None of us are ever far from God whether we are in the best or worst of situations (Psalm 139:7-12). Hiding from God is always a lost cause. We might as well not try.

Emotionally, we may feel close to or far from God; but our emotions are not reliable measures of God's presence. We could feel close to God when we're merely pleased with ourselves, or we could feel far from God because we're lonely or have a poor self-image. First John 3:20 says, "God is greater than our hearts." We can have confidence in God's grace even though our emotions are distressed or confused.

Morally and spiritually, we may be close to or far from God. Some sin, regret, or temptation may be affecting the way we experience our relationship with God. We may be suffering because of the wrongdoing of others, which can make us bitter toward God or desperate for a sense of God's presence.

We could feel close to God because outwardly we are devoted and commendable Christians. Inwardly, however, we may feel disdain, hardness, and hatred toward others instead of the love that the Bible says is indispensable (1 Corinthians 13:1-13; 1 John 4:20).

Believe it or not, we could be far from God because we're too religious! The apostle Paul worried about relying on the Law rather than on faith in Jesus Christ (Galatians 5:4). We can fall away from God's grace by trusting our own religious achievements instead of trusting God's love and initiative.

Perhaps we aren't sure about anything—even about our status with God; but we want to find out more. I've great news for all of us! We are already close to God because of the death and resurrection of Jesus. We don't have to do anything but accept God's love revealed in Jesus and go from there. Jesus has done all the work to bring us close to God— always and for all time—no matter how we feel and no matter what's going on in our lives! That's the wonderful message of the gospel.

Think about all the things you regret, all the things you've done wrong, all the ways you've fallen short over the years. Think of all your most painful secrets and sins. You can think of them, but God does not! Words from the hymn "It Is Well With My Soul" say it well:

My sin, not in part, but the whole
Is nailed to the cross, and I bear it no more.

Certainly regrets and bitter memories require healing, perhaps years of healing. However, as far as your relationship to God is concerned, from God's side, it is settled. Archbishop Desmond Tutu writes, "There is nothing you can do that will make God love you less. There is nothing you can do to make God love you more. God's love for you is infinite, perfect, and eternal."[1] God loves us unreservedly and carries our heaviest burdens.

There's a false notion deeply ingrained in many of us: God will love me only if I'm good enough. Believing in Christ does, indeed, result in a change of heart and life (Romans 6:15-19; 12:1-2); but the things we do as Christians do not earn God's love. When Jesus told his disciples that he was preparing a place for them in his Father's house, he did not tell them to provide all the lumber and the drywall (John 14:1-3). The conditional approval that we experience all around us—in our homes, on our jobs, with our relatives, and with our religious leaders—becomes a model, though a wrong one, for how we perceive God's attitude toward us.

When I was a college student in the mid-1970's, I was shy and hard on myself. I remember how liberating it was to comprehend God's grace and love through Christ. Instead of the erroneous notion that I had to earn God's grace, I felt accepted and chosen by someone who died for me. Of course, I had heard this message all along. I was a lifelong churchgoer, and the gospel of Jesus was familiar to me. I just had not fully comprehended it. God has done more for us than we can imagine; and at different times in our lives, we have to pause and claim for ourselves the wonder of God's grace in Jesus Christ.

For the next few years I explored the life and teachings of Jesus. I didn't yet know how to follow Jesus, and a lot of things in my life still seemed perplexing and unchanged. Using a study Bible and a few good books, I worked my way through the accounts of Jesus' life and studied other parts of the Bible as well. The biblical word *disciple* means "student," so initially I followed Jesus by learning and gaining insights. Hopefully, in this book, I can share the excitement about Jesus that I experienced in college.

I want to focus on the happiness and freedom of the gospel of Jesus. The Scriptures call Jesus many things: Savior, Son of man, Son of God, high priest, rabbi, helper, and friend—among others. The Bible tells us who Jesus is and what he said and did when he walked the earth. The Bible tells us that Jesus still walks with us, and his guidance for each of us continues. God reveals who God is, who we can be, and how we can relate to God and to one another through Jesus.

When Paul preached at the town of Berea in Greece, people were excited about his message of Jesus and began examining "the scriptures every day to see whether these things were so" (Acts 17:11). Let's look at the Scriptures about Jesus with that spirit of joy and expectancy!

Paul Stroble

---

[1] From *Ordinary Graces: Christian Teachings on the Interior Life*, by Lorraine Kisley, editor (Bell Tower, 2000); page 192.

Chapter One

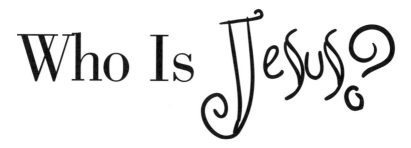

Bible Readings
*Isaiah 9:6-7; Matthew 1–2; 16:13-28; Luke 1–2; Hebrews 4:14–5:10;
Colossians 1:15-20*

The Questions
We have heard of Jesus. We know his name; but who is Jesus, really? What
can we learn about him in the Bible; and how can knowing who Jesus is
make a difference in our lives? In this chapter, you will explore what the
Bible says about the identity of Jesus. Take a moment now and write how you
answer the question "Who Is Jesus?"

_____

_____

_____

_____

_____

_____

_____

A Psalm

I will tell of the decree of the LORD:

He said to me: "You are my son;

today I have begotten you.

Ask of me and I will make the nations your heritage,

and the ends of the earth your possession."

Psalm 2:7-8

A Prayer

Lord, you sent Jesus for us so we can be his precious heritage. Help me learn more about who Jesus is. Teach me how knowing Jesus can make a difference in my life. Teach me to care for Jesus as you care for me and for all the world; in the name of Jesus. Amen.

Something About a Name?

All of us are combinations of different identities and roles. I'm a husband, father, son, friend, teacher, writer, pastor, music lover, cat lover, book collector, fast-food cook (one summer after high school), and so on. Some of our identities are comparatively minor; some are life-long.

What names describe the identities or roles in your life?

REFLECT

Jesus, too, had different identities, names, and ways to understand who he is. All his identities, though, show us God's great love and power! What pops into your head when you hear the name *Jesus*? You might think of names and titles such as *Son of God*, *Messiah*, *Savior*, *Friend*, or *Good Shepherd*. You might think of artistic and media representations: movie depictions of Jesus, da Vinci's *Last Supper*, or Warner Sallman's popular 1941 painting *Head of Christ*, which is found in so many churches. You might even have ambivalent images of Jesus. He's promoted as a quick fix for all your problems, a means to success, and a validation for political positions. When I was a boy, Jesus was "cousin" to Santa Claus. I believed that he knew if I had been bad or good, so I wanted to be good!

The name *Jesus* is an English translation of the Greek *Iesou*s, which in turn comes from the Hebrew *Yeshua*, meaning "the Lord saves." It's the same Hebrew name as *Joshua*, who was a mighty leader in early Israel.

Christ isn't Jesus' last name! It's a title and means the same thing as *messiah*, "anointed one." In ancient times, a new monarch would have fine scented oils poured on his head. As I'll discuss in a moment, the title came to signify a future king who would lead his people. So the usual way we refer to him, "Jesus Christ," is already a statement of who he is.

Jesus' name is no ordinary name. In the first Christian sermon, Peter told the people, "Repent, and be baptized every one of you in the name of Jesus Christ for the forgiveness of your sins; and you will receive the gift of the Holy Spirit" (Acts 2:38). Peter preached that the name *Jesus* would bring about forgiveness and new life. Not long after, Peter told a lame man, "In the name of Jesus Christ of Nazareth, stand up and walk" (Acts 3:6); and the man did so. Peter also told the priestly court, "There is salvation in no one else, for there is no other name under heaven given among mortals by which we must be saved" (Acts 4:12). Jesus' very name connects us to God's great love and power.

3

REFLECT

Bible Facts

The four Gospels (the first four books of the New Testament) give us information about Jesus. Two Gospels, Mark and John, give us nothing about his early life. The other two Gospels, Matthew and Luke, give us stories of Jesus' birth; and Luke gives us the only story of his childhood. All the Gospels give additional space to the last week of Jesus' life—his suffering, death, and resurrection—which alerts us to the importance of those events. The rest of the New Testament—Acts, the Letters, and the Book of Revelation—does not give us biographical material about Jesus; but from that material, we learn things about who Jesus is: Son of Man, Son of God, first-born of creation, high priest, and other names.

BIBLE FACTS

Jesus' Heritage

Ethnically and religiously, Jesus was Jewish. What did Jesus look like? The Bible does not describe him, and no historical accounts exist of his appearance. The December 2002 issue of *Popular Mechanics* published a depiction based on what we know about first-century Semites of that region. The computer-generated face, based on forensics and anthropology, was brown-eyed, darker, and rounder than the auburn-hair, blue-eyed Jesus of so many artistic depictions.[1] Artistic versions of Jesus have varied widely over the centuries.

What do you think Jesus looked like? If you have artistic talent, draw a portrait of Jesus. If you like to write, compose a poem or song lyric about Jesus.

REFLECT

Christians emerge from a wonderful religious tradition, which helps us know the one true God as revealed through the people of Israel (Galatians 4:1-7). Let's honor Jesus by honoring and learning about his people. Ever since Moses, the people of Israel had leaders. Moses led the people to the Promised Land, and then he was succeeded by Joshua. After Joshua, the Israelites were governed by a series of judges. The last judge was named Samuel; and after him, the Israelites had a series of kings, of whom David was the greatest. According to biblical accounts, most of the kings did not follow God's way. The disobedience of the kings and the people were seen as the cause of great misfortune. The Assyrians conquered the northern Israelite kingdom in 722 B.C. The Babylonians conquered the Southern Kingdom in 586 B.C., destroyed the first Temple, and exiled the Hebrews into Babylon for 50 years. (These events are recorded in First Samuel and Second Samuel and First Kings and Second Kings in the Old Testament.)

The prophets spoke God's teachings to the Israelites. Gifted to interpret God's will, they predicted God's punishment falling away from God's laws of justice and mercy; but they also gave the people hope for the future. The prophets looked for a future time when God's righteousness (that is, God's love, justice, and grace) would rule in the land. Some of the prophets looked for a righteous king like David who would represent God's will. The prophets portrayed the king as a giver of justice and righteousness (Isaiah 9:6; 11:2-5), as the establisher of a new covenant (Jeremiah 31:31-34), as a shepherd and servant (Ezekiel 34:23-24), and as a combination of these things (Isaiah 42:6-7; 60:18-19). One prophet predicted that the future king would come from David's hometown (Micah 5:2).

Do you ever have intuitions of things that might happen? If so, what kinds of events do you anticipate?

REFLECT

A Child is Born!
Isaiah 9:6-7

Our first Scripture passage comes from an important prophet who looked to a future king. The previous chapters of Isaiah contain a lot of gloom and doom. Judgment, denunciation, threats, and terrible images predominate. A few light beams of promise shine through, however. Isaiah 2:2-4 promises that God will bring about a time of peace and true worship, and Isaiah 7:10-17 promises the presence of God by the sign of a child named Immanuel, or "God with us." In Chapter 9, God's promise shines through.

What's in the Bible?
Read Isaiah 9:2-7. What words, phrases, or images in this passage speak to you or challenge you? How would this Scripture offer hope to the people of Judah when the threat of Assyrian defeat seemed imminent? How does it help you understand Jesus Christ?

Any period of warfare brings fatigue and discouragement. How long will this conflict go on? How long will a nation suffer oppression? Will peace happen soon? Isaiah 9:2-7 probably dates from the time when the Israelites were under threat from a powerful neighboring kingdom, Assyria. Remember that famous photo of an American sailor hugging and kissing a young nurse when peace was declared in 1945? Peace brings excitement! Some of that excitement can be found in verses 2-5. The bloody and worn-out uniforms can be disposed of, and the people can rejoice.

We could think of other kinds of darkness (verse 2) as well. There is the darkness of depression and sadness; the darkness of sin; the darkness of ruined dreams. "Walking in darkness" is a terrible dilemma; you can't see in the dark, and you're most likely lost.

Isaiah 9:2-7 rests on a promise of what will be. The immediate source of the promise is a new king: the "child born for us." Scholars believe this originally referred to a royal child born in the lineage of David in the late 700's B.C.

Monarchs have titles, often several. The child celebrated in Isaiah is called by several wonderful titles: Wonderful Counselor, Mighty God, Everlasting Father, and Prince of Peace. Further, Isaiah promised that the new king will establish a kingdom of justice, righteousness, and peace. God will bring strength and promise through this child.

Christians have always read these verses as fulfilled in Jesus. Ancient prophecies had meaning for their own time—or near their own time—but some prophecies also became clearer when people centuries later read and interpreted those words. *To fulfill* means "to complete." While Isaiah wrote his divinely inspired words during an earlier era, for Christians, the meaning of these words became complete in Jesus, the Child-King born in the lineage of David.

Isaiah 9:2-7 is often read during the Christmas season.
What insights does it offer you about celebrating the birth of
Jesus Christ?

REFLECT

Newborn Son
Matthew 1–2; Luke 1–2

When I was in high school, my favorite hobby was tracing my family history. I don't have famous relatives, although my great-great-great-grandfather helped build the capitol building in Vandalia, Illinois, where Abraham Lincoln and Stephen A. Douglas served in the legislature. That's my claim to fame. The Gospels of Matthew and Luke give us Jesus' family history (Matthew 1:1-17; Luke 3:23-38). The reading may not seem interesting, but the names are a motley assortment of people. Rahab (verse 5) may be the harlot of Joshua 2:1. Tamar (Matthew 1:3) was the subject of sexual scandal (Genesis 38) as was David himself (Matthew 1:6). Ruth was a Gentile (verse 5), and Manasseh (verse 10) was Judah's worst king (2 Kings 21:1-17). Hezekiah and Josiah were good kings, though. Matthew intended a subtle point: God accomplishes his will in surprising ways through people we might disapprove of from a human point of view—like a pregnant, unwed teenager, which Mary was.

What's in the Bible?

Read the stories of Jesus' birth in Matthew 1–2 and Luke 1–2. What words, phrases, or images in this passage speak to you or challenge you? Which of the stories appeal most to you? Why? What surprises you or makes you want to know more?

Luke's genealogy has a different list of names and also is listed after Jesus' birth. Matthew's Gospel stresses Jesus' Jewish heritage, which is reflected in the genealogy. Luke's writings (the Gospel and Acts) stress the spread of the gospel to the Gentile world; and thus Luke traces Jesus' ancestry all the way back to Adam, the first son of God (Luke 3:38).

Why give a genealogy at all, since according to the accounts in Luke and Matthew, Joseph was not Jesus' father? Jesus' mother was Jewish, though; and through his adoptive (Jewish) father, Jesus was also connected to figures of Israel's history. God's plan has endured through the centuries.

In the stories of Jesus' birth, we learn about the wise men and Herod's villainy from Matthew; and we learn more from Luke's Gospel: the birth of John the Baptist; Mary's pregnancy and her song of praise; the stories of Zechariah, Elizabeth, Simeon, and Anna; and the angels and the shepherds. We also have the well-known story of Joseph and Mary traveling to Bethlehem, lodging in the stable, and placing the newborn Jesus in a manger.

We can pick up significant things implied in the stories. One is certainly the miraculous birth—the mystery of God becoming human. We also see Jesus' family as working people of modest circumstances, but those are the kinds of people he came to help (Luke 1:52-53). Meanwhile, the rulers of the world come and go. We see strong continuities in the birth of Jesus with the traditions of Israel: fulfilled prophecies written hundreds of years before and the hope of God's salvation.

What are your feelings about Christmas? Do you enjoy the season? Do you worry about money for giving gifts? Write down the first things that come to your mind concerning the Christmas season, good and bad. How might the stories of Jesus' birth in Matthew and Luke influence your feelings and thoughts about Christmas?

REFLECT

Son of Man, Son of God
Matthew 16:13-28

I'm guessing that most Christians would call Jesus the Son of God before they'd call him Son of Man. As a kid who went to Sunday school but wasn't otherwise a frequent Bible reader, if I ever heard the term *Son of Man*, I didn't think much about it until I took a college Bible class. We find these two titles for Jesus in Matthew 16:13-28.

What's in the Bible?
Read Matthew 16:13-28. What words, phrases, or images in this passage speak to you or challenge you? What does the phrase Son of Man *say to you about Jesus?* Messiah? Son of the living God?

The term *Son of Man* is used numerous times in Matthew, Mark, and Luke—nearly always in Jesus' own words to refer to himself in the third person. The term can be a euphemism for a human being as is frequently done in the Book of Ezekiel and in Psalm 8. In Daniel 7:13-14 (King James Version), though, "one like a Son of Man" is an otherworldly figure associated with the judgment of God and the end of time.

In this Matthew passage, Jesus puts his friends on the spot. "Who do people say that the Son of Man is?" The disciples gave several possible answers; and then Jesus said, "But who do you say that I am?" You can almost hear them think, *Is this going to be on the quiz?* But Peter supplied the answer, "You are the Messiah, the Son of the living God." Jesus commended Peter's faith and, in fact, promised to build the church upon the "rock" of faith in Christ. The word *messiah* means "anointed," and the Greek word for "messiah" is *Christ*.

Jesus is usually called "Son of God" in the Gospels. For instance, the demons who Jesus exorcised (Mark 3:11; Luke 4:41) recognized him right away. However, others did, too: John the Baptist (John 1:34) and a Roman soldier at the cross (Mark 15:39).

Jesus told his disciples he would have to suffer and die. He associated his own sonship, not with royal privilege or with conquest in the traditional sense but with suffering on behalf of others. Jesus' explanation was unexpected because the messiah was commonly understood to be God's special agent who would vanquish the Romans and reinstate a kingdom of justice and mercy. The messiah was understood as a warrior-king, not as one who would suffer and die.

Read Matthew 16:21-23. What thoughts or feelings do you have about Jesus' response to Peter? What insights does this passage offer to you about Jesus?

REFLECT

Great High Priest
Hebrews 4:14–5:10

Hebrews 4:14–5:10 talks about Jesus as a "great high priest," an image that may be foreign to contemporary ears. The religious system of priests and sacrifices was familiar to those who first read or heard of the Letter to the Hebrews. In many cultures, animals were sacrificed in order to please the gods. In ancient Hebrew society, for example, the shedding of animal blood was a suitable sacrifice demanded by God himself in order that the people's sins would be forgiven. The priest performed such sacrifices on behalf of the people.

What's in the Bible?

Read Hebrews 4:14–5:10. What words, phrases, or images in this passage speak to you or challenge you? What does the phrase great high priest *say to you about Jesus? Read Genesis 14:17-20; Psalm 2:7; 110:4; and Hebrews 7. What insights do these Scriptures offer to the image of Jesus as a "great high priest"?*

For hundreds of years, worship and sacrifices took place in the Temple. The first Temple was built by Solomon in the 900's B.C. and destroyed by the Babylonians in the 500's B.C. A new Temple was constructed later. Jesus and his contemporaries worshiped at this second Temple, but it was destroyed by the Romans in A.D. 70. As the Book of Hebrews notes, the Jewish high priests offered sacrifices in the Temple for God's people (Hebrews 5:1). The priest entered the holiest place of the Temple, the place of God's holy presence. Hebrews 4:14 alludes to that practice of "passing through" the Temple's curtain to enter into God's place, which took place on the Day of Atonement. The priest, who was not sinless, had to make sacrifices for himself in addition to making sacrifices for the people (5:3).

In this Hebrews passage, Jesus himself became God's new high priest who offered himself as the ultimate sacrifice on behalf of the people. He was able to sympathize with human weakness because he was "tested as we are" (4:15). Unlike the levitical priests, however, Jesus was without sin. In addition, Jesus offered himself as the sacrifice. Jesus was presented as an eternal priest "according the order of Melchizedek" (Genesis 14:17-20; Hebrews 5:6, 7).

Some people feel comfortable praying for other people but not for themselves. How do you feel about taking your personal needs and concerns to God? How do you feel about praying for others? How do you feel about others praying for you? What insights do you gain from thinking about Jesus as your great high priest?

REFLECT

The Mystery of Life
Colossians 1:15-20

Colossians 1:15-20 is a beautiful passage that is brimming over with attempts to help people understand the fullness of Jesus' identity in its human and divine aspects. This passage describes Jesus as "the image of the invisible God, the firstborn of all creation." Paul was explaining the significance of Jesus to people who didn't quite understand. Some people thought Jesus was a charismatic moral teacher who died a horrible death. Other people of that time thought Jesus was one of several powerful spiritual beings who came from God. One view emphasized Jesus' human nature, and the other emphasized his divine nature. Paul pointed to Jesus as human and divine.

What's in the Bible?
Read Colossians 1:15-20. What words, phrases, or images in this passage speak to you or challenge you? How do you respond to the idea of Jesus as the "image of the invisible God, the firstborn of all creation"? What insights do you gain from the phrases in him all things hold together *and* in him the fullness of God was pleased to dwell?

In this passage, Paul bridges past, present, and future. First, Jesus is the foundation of all creation. Paul said all things were created through, in, and for him (verse 16). Second, he is the foundation of the universe (verse 17). Christ is fully God and fully part of God's creation.

Bible Facts

We find other names and images for Jesus in the Bible. In John's Gospel, Jesus is called the bread of life (6:35); the good shepherd (10:11); the way, the truth, and the life (14:6); the light of the world and the light of life (8:12), the Word of God (1:1-18), and the resurrection and the life (11:25).

BIBLE FACTS

If you want to know who God is, look at Jesus. If you want to know the secret of the universe, you can also look to Jesus (verse 19).

The phrase *image of God* comes from Genesis 1:26 where God created human beings (Colossians 1:15). Although Genesis 3 tells us that Adam and Eve brought sin into the world, Christ restored humanity to the way God intended. If you want to know what a true human being is like, look to Jesus.

Jesus is the meaning of our future. Jesus brings us eternal life and reconciliation (Colossians 1:18). People needn't struggle to find meaning and die in their sinfulness (verses 18, 20). We find the meaning of all God's purposes, the fullness of God's presence, and all God's power in Jesus.

Who Is Jesus?

We began this chapter with a series of questions: Who is Jesus? How does the Bible name him? How can learning what the Bible says about the identity of Jesus make a difference in our lives?

We hear the name of Jesus so often. Recently I passed a banner in a children's Sunday school wing, "Smile, Jesus loves you!" We hear words like that so often, they start to seem routine, even glib. "Jesus loves me, yada, yada, yada; but I don't feel it, and I need help soon!" As we explore the ways the Bible names Jesus, we begin to see something of God's nature shining through each of the names.

Loving and trusting Jesus is, in many ways, a relationship analogous to our other relationships. We experience love; people who love us validate that love through their words and actions. Love is difficult if our life experiences have hurt us, though, so we have to "keep at it." Likewise, as we grow in Christ's love, we begin to see his love in our life experiences and circumstances. We pray and seek divine help. We stumble sometimes, but we realize God has helped us. We read the Scriptures, and there we find the many ways the Bible names Jesus. We begin to sense that God's nature, revealed through Jesus Christ, is love. We respond by growing in our love and trust of Jesus.

Here's Why I Care

You began this chapter by writing down the ways you answer the question "Who is Jesus?" What would you add to your list after reading the Scriptures in this chapter? How might all the ways of identifying Jesus help you grow in your faith?

HERE'S WHY I CARE

HERE'S WHY I CARE (continued)

A Prayer

Dear God, here's what's going on in my life right now... [Talk to God about your personal situation.] The Bible guides me to you through the many ways it identifies Jesus. Hear my prayer, and guide me in knowledge and awareness of your great love as I continue to explore answers to the question "Who is Jesus?" and allow them to shape my life; in Jesus' name. Amen.

[1]From "Real Face of Jesus," by Mike Fillon in *Popular Mechanics* (December 2002).

Chapter Two

What Did Jesus Say?

Bible Readings
Matthew 5–7; 13:1-52; 22:34-40; 25:31-46

The Questions
In this chapter, you will explore what the Bible says about the teachings of Jesus. What did he teach? Do his teachings continue to have relevance to our lives? What have you heard or what do you remember about the teachings of Jesus?

_____

_____

_____

_____

_____

_____

_____

_____

_____

_____

_____

A Psalm

> Make me to know your ways, O LORD;
>
> > teach me your paths.
>
> Lead me in your truth, and teach me,
>
> > for you are the God of my salvation;
>
> > for you I wait all day long.
>
> > > Psalm 25:4-5

A Prayer

Lord, give me awareness of your will for my life. Help me understand your ways and purposes; in the name of Jesus. Amen.

Jesus the Teacher

My heroes have always been teachers. I am deeply grateful for public school teachers in my past. I'm also grateful for the volunteer teachers in my childhood Sunday school classes. I owe a lot to other teachers who have helped me over the years. One of my best mentors, in fact, was a Reform rabbi in Arizona who encouraged my desire to unite parish ministry with teaching and writing.

One of Jesus' primary activities was teaching. A few times in the Gospels he is called rabbi, which means "teacher" (John 3:2). Modern rabbis lead their synagogue congregations, care for the people, and teach the Hebrew Bible and Jewish traditions.

Jesus traveled the regions of Roman-occupied Palestine, doing good, healing, teaching, and challenging the people. He taught his disciples, individuals whom he encountered, and large groups of people. He taught in synagogues and in the Jerusalem Temple.

What teachers or mentors have been most significant in your life? What did you learn from them? Write about them and about why they meant so much to you in the space provided. Consider writing them a thank-you note.

R E F L E C T

How and with whom did Jesus study? We don't know. What we do know is that by age 12 he wanted to learn from and ask questions of the Jewish teachers at the Temple (Luke 2:41-52). When he began his ministry at the age of 30, he already spoke with authority (Luke 4:22); and his teachings are abundantly recorded in the Gospels.

As we study Jesus' teachings, remember the things we learned in the first chapter about who he is. We risk misunderstanding Jesus' purpose if we see him only as a teacher of principles, even though the principles he taught are excellent guides for everyone throughout all time. Jesus' teachings are intimately connected to his identity as Messiah and Son of God and as our Savior who shed his blood for us and intercedes on our behalf. He continues to love us even when we fail to heed his teachings.

The Kingdom
Matthew 13:1-52

Jesus began his preaching ministry by saying, "Repent, for the kingdom of heaven has come near" (Matthew 4:17), that is, "Turn around! Change what you're doing! Watch out for what God's about to do!" At the opposite end of Matthew, Jesus predicted that God's kingdom would always be preached until the end of time (24:14). What did Jesus mean by the *kingdom of God* (or *kingdom of heaven*)? The Kingdom is an indispensable context for Jesus' teachings. In Chapter 13, Jesus uses several parables as illustrations of the Kingdom.

What's in the Bible?

Read Matthew 13:1-52. What words, phrases, or images in this passage speak to you or challenge you? Which parable appeals most to you? Why?

The Kingdom is God's rule on earth through Christ. Let's call it a spiritual realm of power in the world, the realm where God reigns. To live God's ways of justice, mercy, and love is to participate in God's kingdom now. Christians also look forward with hope to the ultimate reign of God over all creation. People who belong to the Kingdom are those who look to Christ in faith and strive to make him the center of their lives. When you begin to experience Jesus' power in your life, the images of the Kingdom that Jesus used in the parables begin to make sense (Matthew 13:44-45).

Bible Facts

The ancient Israelites considered God their true king, but later God allowed them to have an earthly king to govern them (1 Samuel 8:4-9). One psalm important to early Christians was Psalm 110, which is quoted several times in the New Testament. The psalm shows the Lord giving authority and victory to the messiah king. God even gave the king priestly authority to intercede to God on behalf of people in his governance. Early Christians interpreted this psalm as foreshadowing Jesus.

BIBLE FACTS

In Matthew's Gospel, Jesus likened the Kingdom to sowing seeds. My family comes from rural and agricultural roots; and I love Jesus' images of country living, which derive from the people he knew. The images he used would have been familiar to them. In the parable, a person tossed seed in a field. Birds ate some of the seed. Other seed fell onto bad soil or among thorns and were scorched by the sun or choked by weeds; but some seed fell onto good soil and thus multiplied amazingly (Matthew 13:1-9). The seed grew because of God's power. The soil may refer to those who hear God's word and allow it to grow in their lives.

Jesus also used the images of yeast that causes bread to rise, finding a treasure in a field, and finding a pearl of great value. Each of the images communicates a dimension of truth about God's kingdom. Paul noted that the kingdom of God "depends not on talk but on power" (1 Corinthians 4:20). He understood that the Kingdom is "righteousness and peace and joy in the

Holy Spirit" (Romans 14:17). Paul also taught that God's power results in fruit of the Spirit, which are characteristics of a person who is led by God's power through the Holy Spirit (Galatians 5:22-23).

> *How do you respond to Jesus' use of agricultural images to describe the Kingdom? to the image of the yeast? to finding a treasure or a valuable pearl? What images would you use to describe the Kingdom? Rewrite one of the parables using an image of your own.*

REFLECT

The Sermon on the Mount
Matthew 5–7

When I visited Israel and Palestine, I visited the traditional site of Jesus' Sermon on the Mount. I could easily imagine crowds of people standing or sitting on the side of the large hill in order to hear Jesus.

What's in the Bible?

Read Matthew 5–7. What teachings in this sermon speak to you or challenge you? Which teaching appeals most to you? Why?

With a mountain as the scene, we can make a subtle connection between Moses on Mount Sinai receiving the Ten Commandments, and Jesus on the mount. Jesus taught with the authority of Moses: "You have heard that it was said to those of ancient times. . . . But I say to you. . . ." (Matthew 5:21, 27, 33, 38). The traditions of Moses and of the prophets emphasized love of God and purity of one's heart. If the heart isn't pure, one's religious worship is insincere; and Jesus reaffirmed this emphasis. However, purity of the heart can be more challenging than keeping rules and laws. You could keep your marriage vows inviolate but still be a terrible spouse. You could keep the traffic laws faithfully and still be a self-centered grouch when you drive. For Jesus, devotion involves giving our whole hearts and our whole persons to God and God's way of life. The teachings collected in the Sermon on the Mount set the bar for what it means to live as a member of God's kingdom.

Who Is Blessed?

The Beatitudes are the sayings that begin the sermon (Matthew 5:3-11). *Beatitude* means "blessed" or "happy." In this section, Jesus gives a list of persons who are blessed. What a list! The blessed are those who are spiritually and/or materially needy: the poor in spirit, those who mourn, and the meek. The blessed are those who hunger and thirst for righteousness, the merciful, the pure in heart, the peacemakers, and the persecuted. In effect, Jesus turned the world upside down. We think of happy or blessed people according to different standards.

My daughter and I love to watch *MythBusters* on the Discovery Channel. In an early episode, one of the hosts, when corrected about something he'd said earlier, joked, "I reject your reality and substitute my own." The Beatitudes reject our typical notions of who is successful and happy. We think a happy person is one who has no problems or who has reached closure in a difficult situation. The happy person is self-confident, on top of things. The happy person has planned well and is proud of his or her accomplishments.

Even in our churches we look at worldly models of happiness rather than at Jesus' model. We esteem people with money, power, and influence. We esteem people who are "accomplished" in their faith, who've attended all the right spiritual retreats, who are dynamic speakers and organizers, and who are motivators and attractive personalities.

Maybe we should listen to Jesus and change our expectations about who is blessed or happy. Jesus' "happy people" are the salt of the earth. They preserve the world as salt preserves food and improves its flavor (verse 13). Those who are salt of the earth are also light to the world, bearers of God's own light through their relationship to Christ (verses 14-16).

Difficult Teachings

Some of Jesus' teachings in the sermon seem so difficult (Matthew 5:17-48). When I was little, I was fearful about verse 48: "Be perfect as your heavenly Father is perfect." Is Jesus kidding? He didn't seem like a big kidder. I couldn't even get a volleyball over the net consistently, let alone be perfect like God!

Think of *perfection* as "mature" or "complete," as a holiness of actions and heart. Even the apostle Paul didn't claim to have achieved this (Philippians 3:12-16). Think of Jesus' teachings not as a set of rules that we're supposed to check off when we fulfill them but as commandments that model the kind of love, kindness, and forgiveness that emerge in our lives as a result of our relationship with God.

On our own, we might be able to put away anger so we don't need to retaliate (Matthew 5:21-23, 38-42). Jesus, though, can guide us toward a loving, inner peace plus give us specific circumstances where he knows we can minister in his name. I've no desire to commit adultery; but who hasn't had inappropriate sexual thoughts even if never acted upon? (verses 27-28). Jesus can guide and help us with our sexual needs so we might grow toward purity of heart. I have friends who have experienced the heartache of divorce and who have found new love after the dissolution of a marriage. Jesus spoke about God's will for one loving marriage (verses 31-32), but Jesus is also the loving Savior who helps us through the most difficult circumstances and choices. The challenges of Jesus' teachings continue: Turn the other cheek, give away your cloak, go the second mile, love your enemy. The teachings focus on care for the other no matter who the other happens to be (verses 38-48).

Which of the teachings in Matthew 5:17-48 seem most difficult to you? Why? What would the world be like if everyone practiced these teachings?

REFLECT

Sincere Devotion

Although Jesus wanted our love to be obvious, he didn't want our personal spiritual disciplines to be showy (Matthew 6:1-34). This, too, points back to his concern for a pure heart. Why do we give money to the church? So everyone can know about it? so the pastor will approve of us? because giving is a rule we are obligated to follow? because the love of God in our hearts is expressed naturally and appropriately by giving? Jesus taught that we should give alms (gifts of money or goods) in secret (verses 2-4).

Jesus taught similarly about prayer and fasting (verses 5-18). Most of us pray at one time or other. Perhaps our prayer life is "catch as catch can." Sometimes our prayers are frequent and deep, especially in times of difficulty; but we should never pray for show. Finely worded prayers can be helpful and sincere, but God hears poorly expressed prayers just as readily. He even rushes to help us pray when we've no idea how to express ourselves in words (Romans 8:26).

Some people fast for devotional reasons. If your physician says you can fast without danger to your health (and you do need to ask your doctor), fasting can be a helpful spiritual exercise. The hunger you experience by skipping one or more meals can help focus your attention on God, who supplies our needs. You also become sensitized to the pain experienced by people who are hungry because of poverty. You may become less quick to judge the poor as lazy, deserving of their plight, if you can feel some of their physical needs. In this way, fasting can also help us be less quick to judge others harshly (7:1-5). But, says Jesus, don't go around looking miserable and starved, as if to say, "Look at me, I'm very religious!" How silly! Jesus told people to wash their faces and anoint their heads with oil whenever they fasted. Today he might tell people to freshen up. The idea of spiritual experiences is to draw us closer to God, not to win the approval of people.

Bible Facts

In Isaiah 58, the prophet vividly contrasts true and false worship. The results of any kind of worship and devotion, said the prophet (and Jesus would agree), is to bring the kind of love to other people that meets their needs, changes their lives, and sets them free. Isaiah said choose "to loose the bonds of injustice, / to undo the thongs of the yoke, / to let the oppressed go free" (Isaiah 58:6). The proper fast is "to share your bread with the hungry, and bring the homeless poor into your house" (verse 7). The proper fast involves showing mercy, justice, and compassion.

The Prayer of Jesus

The prayer of Jesus, also known as the Lord's Prayer, captures the essence of living a kingdom life (Matthew 6:8-14). The prayer is so common that we forget to listen to what it says, but it connects the whole of our lives: the holiness of God, the power of God's kingdom, the meeting of our daily needs, our relationship with God, and the purity of our hearts. It begins by naming God's holiness and inviting God's kingdom life to be expressed on earth. In this life, we ask for sustenance one day at a time; we forgive others as God forgives us; and we ask for power that rescues us from evil.

How does the prayer of Jesus speak to you? How might it guide your life?

The prayer of Jesus precedes a challenging teaching about forgiveness (verses 14-15). God will forgive if we forgive, but what if we can't forgive? Some people are hurtful and may be dangerous to our health and well-being. Being forgiving may involve avoiding certain people so we're not in a position to be hurt. Jesus and Paul recognized that you can't be at peace with everyone (Matthew 10:13-14; Romans 12:18). Forgiveness is a process empowered by God that separates persons from actions. It involves perceiving the hurtful person as equally needful of God's love as we are (Matthew 5:43-48). We desperately want God to be forgiving, and God is forgiving; but God also wants us to forgive. At the heart of forgiveness is the profound truth that when we forgive we experience spiritual healing.

Think of people in your life—past or present—that you have a difficult time forgiving. Maybe you don't want to forgive them at all. Talk to God about your feelings; and "cast all your anxiety on him, because he cares about you" (1 Peter 5:7). If you're having difficulty forgiving a certain person, discuss the matter with your pastor or a trusted spiritual guide or a close friend. Write about what might happen if you were able to forgive this person.

REFLECT

Don't Worry

I remember times in my life when money was tight, with no clear solutions ahead. Day-to-day living can be a struggle in those times. Mortgages, college loans, and medical bills can hurt financially. Credit cards provide temporary help; but soon they, too, create a financial emergency. How wonderful we feel when we work through those difficult financial experiences!

Jesus understood the focus on money and called people to "store up . . . treasures in heaven, where neither moth or rust consumes and where thieves do not break in and steal." Money can mislead us from trust in God, "for where your treasure is, there your heart will be also" (Matthew 6:19-21, 24). Misled focus on making money leads to undue anxiety. "Therefore . . . do not worry," Jesus said in the well-known teaching about making a priority the search for God's kingdom and God's righteousness (verses 25-34).

Jesus' teachings apply to all kinds of worry. Anxiety is a well-known concern in contemporary life. Medicines, clinics, and books address the issue. My wife is a calm person who puts trouble in perspective right away, but I tend to slip easily into anxious "what if" thinking. This trait helps make me conscientious about getting things accomplished and helps me avoid procrastination. I have learned that a great way to conquer worry is to address the situation right away, but then I worry when circumstances arise that are out of my control. Jesus taught that we best manage our worry and anxiety by focusing on God and seeking to live God's way. Growing in our trust of God means setting up priorities. We seek first God's kingdom and righteousness (love, mercy, justice, and wisdom) and pray that other aspects of our lives be put into place and cared for by God.

How would you describe yourself in dealing with trouble? (1) cool, calm, and collected; (2) the world's worst worrier; (3) outwardly calm but inwardly anxious; or (4) calm about some things, anxious about others. What difference might it make in your life to make priorities in living your life according to God's way and to seek God's kingdom?

REFLECT

The Great Commandment
Matthew 22:34-40

In one of the college classes I teach, I asked the definition of a *Christian*; and a student replied, "Someone who believes in Jesus and follows the Ten Commandments." I think a lot of Christians would summarize the gospel in that way. I wonder if it would be more accurate to say, "Believe in Jesus and follow the Two Commandments," because Jesus upheld two great commandments: "You shall love the LORD your God with all your heart, and with all your soul, and with all your might" (Deuteronomy 6:5) and "You shall love your neighbor as yourself" (Leviticus 19:18). He taught that these two commandments were at the heart of the Law and the prophets (Matthew 22:40).

What's in the Bible?
Read Matthew 22:34-40. How might this Great Commandment guide your daily decisions and actions?

Jesus understood the heartbeat of God's gift of the Law. In Matthew 5:17, Jesus says, "Do not think that I have come to abolish the law or the prophets; I have come not to abolish but to fulfill." He knew God's law and referred to it frequently.

Read Deuteronomy 6:5 and Leviticus 19:18. Read the Ten Commandments in Exodus 20:1-17. How do you see the commands to love God and neighbor expressed in the Ten Commandments?

REFLECT

You will also find the teaching about the greatest commandment in Mark 12:28-34 and Luke 18:9-14. In Mark and Matthew, Jesus gives the two great commands in response to the lawyer's question. In Luke, Jesus prompts the lawyer to answer and then affirms his response.

Read Matthew 22:34-40; Mark 12:28-34; and Luke 18:9-14. How are they similar? How are they different?

REFLECT

The Least of These
Matthew 25:31-46

Our last reading is one of my favorite passages, and it has inspired and prodded me over the years. Because of these verses, I once took a job teaching classes in prison, which I might not have done otherwise because of my anxiety.

What's in the Bible?

Read Matthew 25:31-46. How do you respond to this Scripture? What words or phrases stand out for you? What challenges you? What inspires you? What prods you?

The teachings in this Scripture occur as one of several teachings Jesus gave in response to the disciples' inquiries about the sign of the Messiah or Son of Man and the end of the age (Matthew 24:3). This passage brings to a logical conclusion all that Jesus taught about what it means to participate in as well as to look forward to God's kingdom, a life in which human action is shaped according to God's power, will, and sovereignty—a life that manifests love of God and neighbor.

Jesus' teachings in the Sermon on the Mount set the stage for all the teachings in Matthew's Gospel. In Matthew 25:31-46, Jesus prepares a kingdom for the blessed. The blessed are those who helped others: gave food to the hungry, clothing to the naked, welcome to the stranger, friendship to the imprisoned. "As you did it to one of the least who are members of my family, you did it to me" (verse 40). He completely identified with the needy, and those who are cast away from Jesus are those who did not serve the needy.

Called to Love

In our churches we celebrate God's salvation offered through Jesus Christ and our decision to accept this gift of grace, and love must result from that grace. We can call Jesus Lord but still be "evildoers," that is, we lack the willingness to love and serve, which is essential for knowing Jesus (Matthew 7:21-23; Ephesians 3:19). In following Jesus, we're called to grow in love and to witness to Christ's love in our everyday circumstances.

Here's Why I Care

Which of Jesus' teachings hold the most meaning for you? Why? In what ways can you practice this teaching during the week ahead?

HERE'S WHY I CARE

HERE'S WHY I CARE (continued)

A Prayer

Dear God, following the teachings of Jesus challenges me. It is not always easy to do what he says. Help me know how best I can hear and practice what he teaches; in Jesus' name. Amen.

Chapter Three

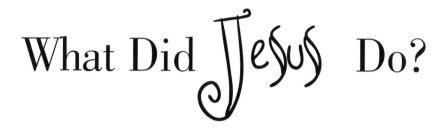

Bible Readings
Matthew 8:1-17; 12:1-14; Mark 5:1-20; Luke 19–24; John 4:1-42; 6:5-14

The Questions
The first four books of the New Testament tell us about Jesus Christ and his ministry. What did Jesus do? How did his life exemplify his identity and his teachings? What do you know or what have you heard about what Jesus did?

_____

_____

_____

_____

_____

_____

_____

_____

_____

_____

_____

A Psalm

> Answer me, O LORD, for your steadfast love is good;
>
> > according to your abundant mercy, turn to me.
>
> Do not hide your face from your servant,
>
> > for I am in distress—make haste to answer me.
>
> Draw near to me, redeem me,
>
> > set me free because of my enemies.
>
> > > Psalm 69:16-18

A Prayer

Lord Jesus, everything you did in your life exhibits God's great love for all. Be with me as I explore what you did and how it can make a difference in my life; in Jesus' name. Amen.

Jesus Reveals God's Love

When we ask, "What did Jesus do?" we look through the lens of Jesus' death and resurrection. Jesus' life and work led him to these events, which are the main focus of the preaching about Jesus that we find in Acts and the New Testament letters. Jesus died and rose again; and through these events, we find salvation, life, hope, and power. However, death and the grave are disturbing, distressing things. What does it mean for God's love to be shown most clearly in events and images that are, from a human standpoint, quite horrible? How did Jesus' actions lead him to the cross? How can we make sense of an empty tomb and resurrection? What Jesus did in his life and ministry—including his suffering, death, and resurrection—demonstrate that God's love went the whole way into human experience. What Jesus did reveals God's love and God's nature. What Jesus did empowers us to be followers of Jesus.

Jesus Healed the Sick

Matthew 8:1-17

Jesus' teachings had characteristics of healing, and his healing miracles had characteristics of teaching. When Jesus taught, he aimed not just at ethical standards but at the healing of our hearts from the disease and power of sin. When Jesus healed people, he not only showed a concern for people's physical needs but also wanted to teach people about God's hope and salvation.

What's in the Bible?

Read Matthew 8:1-17. What thoughts or feelings occur to you as you read these healing stories? What do they say to you about Jesus?

43

In Matthew 8:1-17, we find a series of miracles. First, Jesus healed a man with leprosy. Leprosy, or Hansen's disease, is a chronic and infectious condition that affects the skin, nerves, and respiratory system. The Bible may be referring to that disease or to other kinds of skin maladies, but such maladies involved not only sickness but also social stigma. This man approached Jesus and asked to be made clean. Jesus was not repelled by the man's circumstance and chose to cleanse him (verses 1-4).

When have you felt isolated, avoided, stigmatized, or lonely? What helped you get through the experience?

REFLECT

Jesus also did not begrudge a centurion who approached him for a healing miracle (verses 5-13). A centurion was a Roman soldier who commanded nearly 100 men and was part of the occupying force over a conquered people. He told Jesus that his servant was paralyzed and in distress. Although Jesus offered to come to the soldier's house, the man declined because he believed himself unworthy of Jesus' presence. The soldier told Jesus that he understood Jesus' divine authority because it was analogous to his own authority over his soldiers. Jesus was astounded by the man's faith, especially since the soldier presumably didn't worship the God of the Jews.

Another miracle happened closer to home. Peter was hosting Jesus, but Peter's mother-in-law was ill with a fever. Jesus touched her hand, and she was healed and able to serve a meal (verses 14-17). After these healing stories, Matthew noted that the prophecy of Isaiah was fulfilled in Jesus: "He has borne our infirmities and carried our diseases" (Isaiah 53:4).

Jesus healed several people: the blind (Matthew 9:29-34; Mark 8:22-25; John 9), a woman with a hemorrhage (Mark 5:25-34; Luke 8:43-48)), a paralyzed man (Matthew 9:2-8; Luke 5:18-26), other lepers (Luke 17:11-19), a deaf-mute (Mark 7:31-37), and a woman who couldn't straighten herself (Luke 13:10-17). These healing stories demonstrate Jesus' compassion for those who suffer. They also demonstrate key ideas about Jesus' identity and mission, his power, and his authority. In Luke 13 and John 9, the healings are the source of controversy with some of the religious leaders because they occurred on the sabbath.

It is challenging for us to comprehend the biblical views of healing because the healing stories often involve the miraculous. We have a scientific view of healing that was not part of the biblical view, and we tend to take medical accomplishments for granted rather than view them as miracles. In the biblical view, sickness was associated with sin and evil. It is good to remember that God's healing power may not mean the cure of a disease. Healing may well involve emotional and spiritual aspects of our lives. When we pray for healing for ourselves or our loved ones and the disease remains or death occurs, some Christians may think they did not believe strongly enough or that God was displeased for some reason. Such thinking limits our understanding of God's compassion and care. Stories of Jesus' healings consistently demonstrate God's care and compassion for those who suffer.

Jesus Cast Out Demons
Mark 5:1-20

Jesus cast demons from people, such as the man in Mark 5:1-20. As soon as Jesus began his ministry, he was met by demonic power.

What's in the Bible?
Read Mark 5:1-20. What particularly strikes you about this Scripture? What challenges you or makes you want to know more? What does it say to you about Jesus' power? his identity? his compassion?

Jesus was in a Gentile area, the country of the Gerasenes, east of the Sea of Galilee. As soon as he stepped from the boat, a demon-possessed man came to him. The evil forces present in the man were considerable. The man was so filled with demons that he identified himself as Legion (referring to a Roman legion, which consisted of several thousand men). No one had been able to control him; he was like a monster in a horror story. He even lived in a cemetery! Like the leper and the centurion in the stories we read earlier, Jesus did not disdain the man's needs but addressed his problem.

The demons recognized Jesus and his power immediately. Knowing he was defeated, Legion bargained with Jesus to cast the demons into another living thing—a nearby herd of swine. Perhaps as an ironic comment, Mark wrote that the demons did indeed enter the herd; but that didn't save the evil forces as they hoped, for the swine panicked and killed themselves. Another irony is that swine are unclean animals, which Jews didn't consider proper to raise or eat; and Jesus rid the area not only of demons but of an animal whose meat was forbidden for Jews. The non-Jewish herdsmen were understandably upset at the loss.

Bible Facts

Several biblical stories deal with the reality of evil personified in Satan or the devil. First Peter 5:8 cautioned people to be watchful because "like a roaring lion your adversary the devil prowls around, looking for someone to devour." However, Peter promised that we can stand firm in our faith and resist him. Elsewhere in the Bible we learn that Jesus was tempted directly by Satan (Matthew 4:1; Luke 4:2). Revelation 20 tells us that Satan will be subdued for a thousand years and then defeated forever; but in the meantime, the death and resurrection has dealt the devil a mortal blow (John 12:31-32; 16:33). Stories of Jesus' exorcisms show the reality of evil and his power over evil and death, a power revealed in his resurrection.

BIBLE FACTS

Notice that the man received a new mission. Jesus declined to have the man follow him but gave him an alternative: Jesus told him to spread the news among his own people that God had shown him mercy. The demoniac became one of the first Gentile preachers about the power of Jesus. Stories such as this remind us that evil does not have the last word even as much as we may suffer in this life.

How do you understand evil? In what way does God's power over evil make sense to you? How do you explain the persistence of evil in our world

R
E
F
L
E
C
T

Jesus Fed the Multitude
John 6:1-14

In John 6:1-14, Jesus feeds 5,000 people with one person's food; and several baskets of food are left over. The feeding of the 5,000 is the only miracle of Jesus (besides the Resurrection) that is recorded in all four Gospels (Matthew 14:13-21; Mark 6:30-44; Luke 9:10-17; John 6:1-14).

What does this miracle mean for us today?

R
E
F
L
E
C
T

What's in the Bible?

Read John 6:1-14. What images, words, or phrases grab your attention, challenge you, or make you want to know more? What does this passage say to you about Jesus? about the disciples? about the 5,000?

One of the wonderful results of Bible reading, gained over time, is the ability to make connections among stories and verses. During the time of Moses, God gave special food called manna to the Israelites in order to sustain them (Exodus 16:4-21). In that story, too, God fed several thousand people who had insufficient food. The Gospel miracle is a sign that God was gathering a people and sustaining them.

The prophet Elisha's feeding of 100 people with 20 barley loaves and fresh ears of grain (2 Kings 4:42-44) also parallels the story of the feeding of the 5,000. Elisha asked a man from Baal-shalishah to distribute the food; and miraculously, the people had enough to eat. They also had leftovers.

These stories demonstrate God's power and God's compassion for the hungry. Such compassion was demonstrated in the early church. James 2:15-17 reads, "If a brother or sister is naked and lacks daily food, and one of you says to them, 'Go in peace; keep warm and eat your fill,' and yet you do not supply their bodily needs, what is the good of that? So faith by itself, if it has no works, is dead." Jesus gave the crowd words, but he also met their physical needs.

Bible Facts
An important part of Christian worship is the Lord's Supper, also called the Eucharist or Holy Communion. In this ritual, Christians share bread and wine or grape juice. The bread represents Jesus' body. The wine or grape juice represents Jesus' blood (Luke 22:14-20; 1 Corinthians 11:23-26). The act of worship recalls and proclaims Jesus' sacrificial love. The rite is a sacrament (a church practice by which God provides grace). The ritual helps Christians remember, offer thanks, and experience togetherness as the community of believers.

BIBLE FACTS

Jesus Broke Down Social Barriers
John 4:1-42
Jesus caused controversy in part because he broke down social barriers as he reached out to people.

What's in the Bible?

Read John 4:1-42. How do you respond to this story? What especially strikes you about the conversation between Jesus and the Samaritan woman? What does Scripture say to you about Jesus? about the woman? about the Samaritans who proclaimed that Jesus was Savior of the world?

In John 4, Jesus struck up a conversation with a Samaritan woman. When Jesus asked the Samaritan woman for a drink of water, he broke two social taboos. During the time of Jesus, relationships between Jews and Samaritans were strained (verse 9). The disciples were "astonished that he was speaking with a woman" (verse 27), because it was a breach of propriety for Jewish men to speak to women in public. Yet, not only did Jesus ask the Samaritan woman for water, he engaged in conversation with her. As a result of the conversation with the woman and her witness to her neighbors, the Samaritans asked Jesus to stay. He preached to them for two days, and they believed that Jesus was the "Savior of the world" (verses 40-42).

Bible Facts

Samaritans were originally the people who lived in what became the northern kingdom of Israel. In 721 B.C., the Assyrians conquered Israel and displaced many of the people. Many of those who remained then intermarried with Assyrian captives who were brought in from other conquered regions. In 587 B.C., Jerusalem was conquered by the Babylonians; and most of the leading citizens were exiled. When Ezra and Nehemiah were allowed to return to Jerusalem to rebuild the Temple and the wall, they refused to allow the Samaritans to help (Ezra 4:1-3; Nehemiah 4:7). These and other events contributed to the long-standing animosity between Jews and Samaritans that was evident during the time of Jesus.

BIBLE FACTS

Other episodes in the Gospels demonstrate Jesus breaking down barriers between Jews and Samaritans. Jesus criticized the disciples for their hostility to the Samaritans (Luke 9:55-56), healed a Samaritan leper (17:16), honored Samaritans with a story demonstrating neighborliness (10:30-37), and commended a Samaritan for his gratitude (17:11-19). Jesus helped Zacchaeus, who was a social outcast because he collected taxes for the Romans. His life had been scarred by greed. The company of Jesus helped Zacchaeus change his life and make up for his past (19:1-10). Still another is the story of the Canaanite woman who approached Jesus for an exorcism miracle. Jesus seemed to dismiss her harshly; but she persisted and answered him cleverly, displaying an amazing faith (Matthew 15:21-28).

Ephesians 2 emphasizes Jesus' barrier-breaking work as it talks about Jewish and Gentile followers of Jesus in the early Christian community: "For he is our peace; in his flesh he has made both groups into one and has broken down the dividing wall, that is, the hostility between us" (2:14). Through his death and resurrection, Jesus has removed all the barriers that we persist in raising (verses 14-22).

How does Jesus breaking barriers speak to contemporary life? What social or cultural barriers do you see in our world? What hope does Jesus offer for breaking such barriers?

REFLECT

Jesus Challenged Religious Leaders
Matthew 12:1-14

Though Jesus consistently pointed to God's compassion, mercy, and justice over and above unreasonable interpretations of the Law, his actions angered religious leaders. Matthew 12:1-14 focuses on Jesus' willingness to violate sabbath laws.

What's in the Bible?
Read Matthew 12:1-14. How do you respond to Jesus' actions in this passage? Why do you think religious leaders became so angry with Jesus?

Jesus often spoke angrily to the leaders of his time, and he challenged the status quo. We shouldn't think of his teachings as non-Jewish or anti-Jewish nor of his anger as prejudice, however. Jesus' anger arose from his concern for people's well-being, just as you and I become angriest at those we love. Jesus and all his friends, family, and disciples were Jewish. Like other rabbis, he stressed the centrality of Leviticus 19:18 and Deuteronomy 6:4 among the many Old Testament commandments (Matthew 22:34-40). Jesus taught the meaning of the Jewish law and the prophets according to his own authority (Matthew 5:17-20; John 1:17). In John's Gospel, he places himself at a level of intimacy with God that seemed blasphemous (John 5:17-18).

We might say, "Well, of course he did; he's Jesus!" However, we have hindsight for understanding Jesus. After the Jews returned from their 50-year exile in Babylon as recorded in the books of Ezra and Nehemiah, they rebuilt Jerusalem and the Temple and re-established their religious life. According to Bible scholar Suzanne de Dietrich, "For this tiny remnant of Israel, the only ones who had survived disaster, faithfulness means specific obedience to God's commandments. This involves an attachment to ceremonies and institutions that to us today may seem outdated, but that then were the only means of safeguarding religious integrity."[1] Jesus' critics perceived him as a danger to the faithfulness of his own people.

Another difficulty was the threat of Roman crackdown. The occupying Roman forces typically insisted that conquered peoples honor the Roman emperor as a god. The Jews would not do so, and so Rome made an exception in their case. However, someone such as Jesus, who was considered a potential king of the Jews, might have caused enough tension among the Romans that they would crack down on the Jews—as the Romans indeed did about 40 years later when they destroyed the Jerusalem Temple.

How do you think Jesus might challenge the status quo of our culture? Who are those in our history who have challenged injustice or lack of mercy?

REFLECT

Jesus Suffered, Died, and Rose From the Dead
Luke 19–24

Recently I visited the college that my daughter plans to attend, a Roman Catholic school with an interdenominational student body. As is typical in Catholic churches and schools, the crucifix—an artistic representation of Jesus nailed to the cross—is a common sight. I noticed a large one in the dining hall. The cross is a powerful symbol of God's love through Christ.

To understand why Jesus' death is an expression of love, try this "thought experiment." Pretend that you know nothing about Christianity. You enter the main gathering room of a group of happy people, and on the wall is a representation of a human corpse. The dead person was abused prior to death, and the body wasn't even made presentable for respectful funeral viewing. How could a dead body be a symbol of love, an appropriate centerpiece for a room?

You could similarly look afresh at the meaning of Jesus' resurrection. If you're walking through a cemetery and encountered a dug-up grave and the burial vault open, you wouldn't think, *A resurrection has happened.* You'd assume the body had been disinterred; but why? What happened?

What's in the Bible?
Read about the last days of Jesus' life on earth, his crucifixion, and his resurrection in Luke 19–24. How do you respond to the events described in Luke? What scenes particularly stand out for you? Why?

56

All four Gospels have similar accounts of Jesus' last week. He entered Jerusalem, cleansed the Temple, and taught the people. He discussed the end times with his disciples. Behind the scenes, the religious leaders plotted his death and enlisted one of Jesus' disciples to help them. Jesus had a last supper with his disciples, specifically the Jewish Passover meal. Later that evening, he went to an area of olive trees called Gethsemane to pray. There, Jesus was arrested. While Jesus was in custody, Peter denied knowing him. Jesus was examined by the religious leaders and then by the Roman governor Pontius Pilate, who ordered him crucified.

Crucifixion was a Roman means of execution—essentially death through torture, whereby the condemned person was nailed or tied naked to a crossbeam of wood and suspended upright. Death came through asphyxiation due to strain on the lungs as the body hung for hours and sometimes days. A victim could also die of shock from the trauma of scourging if the victim was whipped prior to crucifixion. The execution not only involved prolonged pain but it was also degrading. The condemned person helplessly suffered the scorn of onlookers. Death could be hastened by breaking the victim's legs (creating internal bleeding and trauma) or by lancing the victim with a spear. Jesus died after six hours of crucifixion. He was speared in the side prior to being removed from the cross.

Bible Facts

The prophet Isaiah wrote about the suffering servant (42:1-4; 49:1-6; 50:4-9; 52:13–53:12.) We're not sure whom Isaiah intended for this image to represent: apparently not a king, but perhaps the Israelites personified another prophet. For Christians, this image is fulfilled in Jesus. Isaiah 52:13–53:12, in particular, speaks of a person horribly abused and punished but whose sufferings brought healing power to many people. These writings predate Jesus by several centuries.

BIBLE FACTS

After all this hideous and inhumane treatment, Jesus was given a respectful burial. The Jewish leader Joseph of Arimathea (and, according to John's Gospel, also the Jewish leader Nicodemus) prepared the body. Joseph of Arimathea had an unused tomb in which he placed the body of Jesus.

Jesus' disciples were nowhere on the scene (imagine yourself dying and your closest friends avoid you), but several women had stayed with Jesus and intended to anoint the body. When they arrived at the tomb, they discovered that it was empty. The risen Jesus appeared to Cleopus and a friend on the road to Emmaus and to the disciples. He reminded them what he had taught them: "Thus it is written, that the Messiah is to suffer and to rise from the dead on the third day, and that repentance and forgiveness of sins is to be proclaimed in his name to all nations, beginning from Jerusalem" (Luke 24:46-47). Then Jesus made a promise to them: "And see, I am sending upon you what my Father promised; so stay here in the city until you have been clothed with power from on high" (verse 49).

Life and Power Through the Resurrection

Everything Jesus did culminated in the gifts of life and power given to us through the Resurrection. Christians are a resurrection people. Jesus is more fully present than ever before through the power of the Spirit. Not only do we see our potential for acting and doing when we look at what Jesus did in his earthly ministry, we have God's power to do what God calls us to do in Jesus' name.

Here's Why I Care

How do Jesus' actions speak to you? How do you feel about his healing? his power over evil? his challenges to the religious authorities of his day? his breaking down social barriers? his crucifixion and resurrection? the promise of God's power through the Spirit? How might any or all of these actions influence your life?

HERE'S WHY I CARE

HERE'S WHY I CARE (continued)

A Prayer

God of life and resurrection, thank you for showing your love, mercy, power, and salvation through all that Jesus did. Help me be more like Jesus in my actions; in Jesus' name. Amen.

---

[1]From *God's Unfolding Purpose: A Guide to the Study of the Bible*, by Suzanne de Dietrich (The Westminster Press, 1974); page 137.

Chapter Four

How Can We Respond to Jesus?

Bible Readings

Matthew 28:18-20; Luke 15:11-32; John 15:1-17; 16:19-24; 17:10-13;
1 Corinthians 12:12-27; Ephesians 4:1-16

The Questions

The life, ministry, crucifixion, and resurrection of Jesus reveal and demonstrate God's amazing love for us. How can we respond to God's self-giving love in Jesus Christ? What thoughts or feelings do you have about what Jesus did? What difference can it make in our lives and in the lives of others?

_____

_____

_____

_____

_____

_____

_____

_____

_____

_____

A Psalm

Praise the LORD!

I will give thanks to the LORD with my whole heart,

in the company of the upright, in the congregation.

Great are the works of the LORD,

studied by all who delight in them.

Full of honor and majesty is his work,

and his righteousness endures forever.

Psalm 111:1-3

A Prayer

God of power and life, help me see your will for my life as I explore ways I can respond to Jesus; in his name I pray. Amen.

Visiting Your House Today?

When I was a child, my second/third-grade Sunday school class learned about Zacchaeus, a small man and a hated tax collector who climbed a tree to see Jesus over the crowds. Jesus noticed him, perceived something deeper in his curiosity, and invited himself to Zacchaeus's house. Soon Zacchaeus told Jesus how he was going to turn his life around (Luke 19:1-10).

A Sunday school teacher asked us, "What if Jesus came to your house?" For one thing, my mother would have panicked! She worried about the condition of our house, especially as careless as Dad could be with his stuff. If Jesus had come to our house, I doubt he would have commented on house-keeping skills. Jesus always helped people to learn and grow. He helped to heal and guide them. Everything we know about him pertains to his life and work for us. It is more challenging to consider what we might want to do for Jesus and to consider how we can respond to his love for us.

Accept God's Love
Luke 15:11-32

When some of the Pharisees and scribes grumbled because Jesus welcomed such disreputable people as tax collectors and scribes, Jesus told a parable about a man and his two sons. It is a classic story of God's love and the willingness or lack of willingness to accept it.

What's in the Bible?

Read Luke 15:11-32. What is your response to this story? Which son gains your greatest empathy and understanding? Why? How do you respond to the father of the two sons? What does this story say to you about God's love?

63

The younger son's actions were reprehensible. He demanded his inheritance and chose an excessive lifestyle that was different from what was expected from a faithful Jew. When he lost all his money, he "came to himself" and decided to return home, confess his sin, and ask to be among his father's hired hands (Luke 15:17). His father saw him coming, ran to him, put his arms around him, kissed him, and prepared a homecoming celebration. This would have been a joyous end to the story, but the elder brother became angry. He refused to go in and told his father, "Listen! For all these years I have been working like a slave for you, and I have never disobeyed your command; yet you have never given me even a young goat so that I might celebrate with my friends. But when this son of yours came back, who has devoured your property with prostitutes, you killed the fatted calf for him" (verses 29-30). The father offered love and grace to the elder son: "Son, you are always with me, and all that is mine is yours. But we had to celebrate and rejoice, because this brother of yours was dead and has come to life; he was lost and has been found" (verses 31-32). Jesus' story is open-ended. Would the elder son accept the father's love and in so doing embrace and welcome his brother?

How do you think the elder brother might respond? Why? Do you think the situation is fair to the elder son? Why or why not? What do the father's words to him say to you about God's love?

REFLECT

Many of us have a difficult time comprehending and accepting the completely free love of God illustrated in Jesus' parable. We think that we need to do something to earn it. We need to be good, to be honest, to love people. True, those things are important; but God loves us whether we've lived good or despicable lives! Yet we might be uncertain about God's love for us. We worry that God will reject us. What if we have done 9,999 good things in our lives but 10,000 wrong things? Will God reject us just because we are two good deeds short of a majority? No, that kind of thinking is all wrong; it puts the emphasis upon our imperfect works instead of God's love and initiative. Why would Jesus die and rise if our salvation were based on our imperfect efforts?

Have you ever thought or felt that God's love for you depends upon what you do? How do you understand doing good in relation to God's love for you? Can you think of anyone in history whose actions challenge the belief that God loves everyone?

REFLECT

Paul understood that "we all have sinned and fall short" (Romans 3:23). In Romans 5:1-18 and Galatians 5:1, he speaks about salvation as a free gift offered through faith in Christ. If we understand Paul's main point, the letter becomes a wonderful call to freedom. Paul emphasized that we can do nothing to guarantee our salvation because God has done everything we need through Jesus Christ. God has even made it possible for us to know we're saved. As believers, we experience the power of the Holy Spirit. We're set free from any compulsion to please God through our own efforts and achievements. In that freedom, we have life, joy, and power to serve others.

> *How do you respond to the message that God's love in Christ is a free gift? How does it feel when you accept a gift from someone? What connections do you make between accepting a gift and accepting the love of God in Jesus Christ?*

REFLECT

Abide in Jesus
John 15:1-9

The way to grow in love of God and neighbor is to abide in Christ. *Abide,* which has the sound of an old-fashioned word, means "to wait patiently" or "to remain in a place for a while." This sense of staying, remaining, and being present is expressed when Jesus said to the disciples, "Abide in me as I abide in you" (John 15:4).

What's in the Bible?

Read John 15:1-9. How do you respond to the image of Jesus as a vine and God as the vine grower? What does it say about being in relationship with Jesus Christ?

I had a good friend who raised grapes in his backyard. He was an elderly man who liked to work with vines and prune plants and coax the grapes to ripeness. He gave away most of his crop to neighbors and friends, including my father, who, in turn, used the grapes to make jelly and gave my friend some. In John 15:1-5, Jesus likened himself to a vine and the disciples to the branches. He told the disciples to abide in the vine and thus bear fruit. In other words, remaining in relationship with God through Jesus Christ makes discipleship possible.

As we explored earlier, our good works do not earn God's love and salvation. They emerge from our relationship with God through Christ. Becoming a fruit-bearing Christian is a lifelong journey. The image of the vine, the branches, and the vine grower communicates that the power to bear fruit in our lives comes from God. Fruit bearing is the capacity to keep the commandments and remain in the love of God through Christ (verse 10).

How does fruit bearing apply to your life? How might a deeper relationship with God through Jesus Christ empower your life?

REFLECT

Jesus noted that God prunes the branches that they might bear more fruit (verse 2). The image of pruning implies pain and loss, and tragedies and disappointments sometimes strike us as painful and senseless. We should be careful not to think that all trouble in our lives comes from God. Trouble, though, can help us draw closer to God. Romans 8:28 teaches that God is present in all life circumstances and brings good from them. If life steers us toward new beginnings, we can take the opportunity to ask God what directions we should pursue. Though change can be painful, we can be assured that God wills good in our lives.

Have you ever thought that God eliminated or pruned something in your life? How did you feel? What was the result?

REFLECT

Love Others
John 15:10-17

I remember how the word *love* was in the air in the 1960's and 1970's. Seemingly, most of the musical groups sang songs about love. A popular novel in 1970 was *Love Story*. People flocked to music festivals and celebrated love. Love is a good thing. It continues to be a major theme of books, music, television, and movies; but it is often tossed around lightly. Its meaning is too frequently limited to emotion, romance, and physical attraction. Love as Jesus taught goes much deeper than, and frequently is different from, an emotional feeling.

What's in the Bible?

Read John 15:10-17. How do you understand love? What does this Scripture say to you about the way Jesus understood love?

In Chapter 2, we looked at the two great commandments that Jesus referred to in what we now call the Great Commandment (Matthew 22:34-40; Mark 12:28-34; Luke 10:25-28). Deuteronomy 6:4 says, "Hear, O Israel: The LORD is our God, the LORD alone. You shall love the LORD your God with all your heart, and with all your soul, and with all your might." The affirmation of God's reality is included with a call to love God with your whole self, no matter what. What does it mean to love God with the heart? The biblical word *heart* has a broader meaning than just our emotional feelings. The word also means a lot more than the muscle in our chests. In the Bible, *heart* is a metaphor for our whole selves: our minds, will, emotions, and affections. We can feel good about God, but feeling good does not quite capture the whole meaning of loving God.

In Leviticus 19:18, "You shall love your neighbor as yourself: I am the LORD," the word *love* is again closely associated with the reality of God. You may be able to love other people without loving God, but it is almost impossible to love God without loving other people. First John 4:19-21 cautions us that if we do not love brothers and sisters whom we see, then we can't love God whom we haven't seen.

Consider memorizing the two great commandments, or write them down and place them on your bathroom mirror or some other place where you see them daily. Practice keeping these commandments in mind so you will be aware of them as you go about your daily business. How do you think this practice might affect your daily life?

REFLECT

When we are in a loving relationship, we want to do things with and for that person. We can think of our relationship to God through Jesus Christ in that way. While we don't have to worry about God's love for us, we demonstrate our love for God through our actions. Do we expect people to tolerate our grumpy moods without complaint? Do we prefer being with the "right" people? Do we judge others of different ethnic or social groups? Doesn't God accept us just as we are? Yes. God does. We don't earn or win God's love. However, one of the joys of salvation is to experience God's cleansing of our faults, blind spots, and sins. We experience God's power to transform us into people who are capable of loving. Paul speaks of being "transformed by the renewing of your mind, so that you may discern what is the will of God—what is good and acceptable and perfect" (Romans 12:2). We hear people talk about "seeking God" in order to find peace and meaning. When we seek God through relationship with Jesus Christ, we will be changed. We will see in our lives the fruit of the Spirit: kindness, gentleness, patience, peace, love, joy, self-control, generosity, and faithfulness (Galatians 5:22-24). We learn to trust God even when life seems dark and terrible. We experience God's gifts of renewal and holiness. We learn to accept that God loves all people and that we can be empowered to love.

How do you feel about or what do you think about the idea that God could transform or change you? What difference might God's transformation make in your life? Do you think you would be the same person? Why or why not? What might God change in your life?

REFLECT

Teach Others About Jesus
Matthew 28:16-20

Christians call Matthew 28:16-20 the Great Commission. It contains Jesus' instruction to his followers to make disciples, to baptize, and to teach obedience to all that Jesus taught.

What's in the Bible?
Read Matthew 28:16-20. What challenges you about this Scripture? What in the passage offers hope?

The Great Commission seems to focus on what Christians traditionally call witnessing, that is, to tell about Jesus and encourage others to become part of the Christian faith. Certainly, this is an aspect of the passage; but the message of this commission is deeper and more complex. It has everything to do with the formation of communities of believers who practice and teach the way of Jesus. Even though some disciples still doubted, they were entrusted with the mission (Matthew 28:17). We see that Jesus has been given all authority in heaven and on earth (verse 18). The Baby, who was worshiped by non-Jewish wise men in Matthew 2 and who grew up to be crucified and mocked as "king of the Jews" in Matthew 27, had become the risen Christ who reigns over God's present and coming realm for all time. The risen Christ commissions the worshiping and doubting disciples to "make disciples of all nations." All people from all nations are invited to become followers of Jesus and to put into practice what Jesus taught. Baptism brings them into discipleship within this community. As part of functioning and active Christian communities, disciples are commissioned to teach all that Jesus taught. What the Great Commission reveals is the essential nature of the church over which Jesus Christ reigns. The Great Commission calls each one of us and all of us to teach and live the way of God's kingdom, a way that was taught and lived by Jesus Christ.

Bible Facts

In Matthew 28:19, the Greek word *matheteuo* is translated "make disciples" in the New Revised Standard Version of the Bible and "teach" in the King James Version. The word in Greek is a verb, and it means "to instruct" or "to teach." In the noun form, the word *disciple* essentially means "student" or "learner."

BIBLE FACTS

As individuals who participate in communities of faith, we are disciples of Jesus Christ, which means we are always learning and growing. We are likewise helping others to learn and grow through our words and through our actions. While Christians honor and serve Jesus Christ, we get lost when we insist that our experiences should be normative for others. The God who created us and who offers hope and life in Jesus Christ recognizes and celebrates our variety.

How do you see the Great Commission at work in church? in the lives of individual Christians you know? How do you think you might respond to the Great Commission?

REFLECT

Be Part of the Body of Christ
1 Corinthians 12:12-27; Ephesians 4:1-16

Earlier in the chapter we looked at John 15 and the image of a vine and its branches. Jesus' words about the vine and branches are not at all individualistic. We grow because we are connected to Jesus; however, lots of other branches are connected to Jesus as well. "Solitary Christian" is an oxymoron. Jesus wants us to be together. Paul put it another way when he talked about life in the early Christian communities as the body of Christ.

What's in the Bible?
Read 1 Corinthians 12:12-27 and Ephesians 4:1-16. How does the image of Christians as the body of Christ speak to you? What does it say to you about the way people can function together as a community of individuals who follow Jesus Christ?

We all know that our body parts work together. For example, if my back hurts, my whole body slows down. Similarly, when the church functions well as Christ's body, all the parts—pastors, teachers, musicians, administrators, worshipers, and others—work together and do not disdain one another's gifts. If one group is in turmoil, however, the whole church is affected; or if a few faultfinders start to spoil things, negativity spreads throughout the congregation.

I dearly love churches. I'm in my fifties and have been part of churches my whole life—since the days I was a kid in Sunday school and vacation Bible school. Sometimes our churches fail to communicate the gospel in a way that helps others. We attend a church and discover that it has cliques and in-groups. We don't experience God's love because we're not in and we don't know how to get in. We come to church desperately seeking God's love, but that week the pastor is sternly preaching about righteous living and accountability. We may feel scolded and inadequate. We attend church to find God; and we are hit by a list of committees to volunteer for, pledge cards for financial giving, and people eager to get our addresses and phone nubers.

What have been your experiences of churches? Have you felt welcomed at churches you've attended? Have you felt annoyed or hurt at something?

REFLECT

In a sincere desire to help our congregations grow, develop, and be healthy, church leaders unintentionally send the signal that the Christian life is a list of dos, don'ts, have-tos, and programs, rather than a wonderful, joyful response to God's overwhelming love revealed in Jesus Christ. Churches are frail human places, but churches are also wonderful places of grace where people care for you.

All the churches named in the New Testament had issues and challenges of various kinds. Paul recognized that when people who believe in Christ came together as worshiping communities, many God-given gifts graced the community. We are part of the body of Christ when we honor our own gifts and the gifts of others as we offer them to the service of Christ. We need each other in order to offer the hope and love of Jesus Christ to everyone.

What talents and skills do you have that you might offer to the church? How might offering your talents and skills enrich your life? the life of the church?

REFLECT

Paul noted that the church works well when everyone aims at maturity, "to the measure of the full stature of Christ" (Ephesians 4:13). People help one another grow and develop in Christ; they help one another believe rightly; and they teach and assist one another in the work of ministry. Christian growth always presupposes growth alongside other growing Christians. Our growth, in turn, helps transform the church into a body built up in love, truth, and maturity.

Claim the Joy of Christ
John 16:19-24; 17:10-13

In John 16:19-24, Jesus encourages the disciples who would soon have to continue without his human presence. He promised them that they would know joy that no one would be able to take away from them (16:22). In John 17:10-13, Jesus prays that the joy he had known would be made complete in the disciples.

What's in the Bible?
Read John 16:19-24; 17:10-13. How do you understand joy?
What causes you to experience joy? What do you think Jesus
meant by joy *in these passages?*

I'm often amazed at how many times Scriptures tells us not to be afraid. In Luke 2:10, the angels tell the shepherds, "Do not be not afraid; for see, I am bringing you good news of a great joy." In Matthew 28:10, Jesus tells the disciples, "Do not be afraid." In Luke 24:38-39, Jesus tells the disciples, "Why are you frightened, and why do doubts arise in your hearts? Look at my hands and my feet; see that it is I myself." In John 20:19, 26, Jesus declares, "Peace be with you." In John 14:27, Jesus says, "Do not let not your hearts be troubled, and do not let them be afraid." In John 15:11, Jesus says, "I have said these things to you so that my joy may be in you, and that your joy may be complete." Jesus understood that ultimate and complete joy, something profoundly deeper than a simple emotional response to a happy situation, emerged from living in relationship with God. This joy persists through heartbreak, loss, or any situation that may cause pain in our lives.

Respond to God's Love for You

Joy, peace, and freedom from fear come from God's love for us in Jesus Christ. No matter what else is going on in our lives, that love is constant and unending. "If God is for us, who is against us?. . . For I am convinced that neither death, nor life, nor angels, nor rulers, nor things present, nor things to come, nor powers, nor height, nor depth, nor anything else in all creation, will be able to separate us from the love of God in Christ Jesus our Lord" (Romans 8:31, 38-39). Such unending love calls for our response.

Here's Why I Care

Make a list of your talents. What are they? How can you use them to respond to the love God gives you through Jesus? to communicate God's love in Jesus Christ to others? What one thing can you do in the next few days?

HERE'S WHY I CARE

HERE'S WHY I CARE (continued)

A Prayer

Thank you, God, for the gift of your love through Jesus Christ. Help me discover how I can use the gifts you have given me in order to serve him. Give me a hunger to understand more. Give me a passion to show love to other people in Jesus' name. Help me know for myself the joy of Christ. Amen.

APPENDIX

PRAYING THE BIBLE

Praying the Bible is an ancient process for engaging the Scriptures in order to hear the voice of God. It is also called *lectio divina*, which means "sacred reading." You may wish to use this process in order to become more deeply engaged with the Bible readings offered in each chapter of this study book. Find a quiet place where you will not be interrupted, a place where you can prayerfully read your Bible. Choose a Bible reading from a chapter in this study book. Use the following process to "pray" the Bible reading. After you pray the Bible reading, you may wish to record your experience in writing or through another creative response using art or music.

Be Silent

Open your Bible, and locate the Bible reading you have chosen. After you have found the reading, be still and silently offer all your thoughts, feelings, and hopes to God. Let go of concerns, worries, or agendas. Just *be* for a few minutes.

Read

Read the Bible reading slowly and carefully aloud or silently. Reread it. Be alert to any word, phrase, or image that invites you, intrigues you, confuses you, or makes you want to know more. Wait for this word, phrase, or image to come to you; and try not to rush it.

Reflect

Repeat the word, phrase, or image from the Bible reading to yourself and ruminate over it. Allow this word, phrase, or image to engage your thoughts, feelings, hopes, or memories.

Pray

Pray that God will speak to you through the word, phrase, or image from the Bible reading. Consider how this word, phrase, or image connects with your life and how God is made known to you in it. Listen for God's invitation to you in the Bible reading.

Rest and Listen

Rest silently in the presence of God. Empty your mind. Let your thoughts and feelings move beyond words, phrases, or images. Again, just *be* for a few minutes. Close your time of silent prayer with "Amen"; or you may wish to end your silence with a spoken prayer.